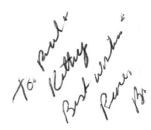

LIVING WITH PARKINSON'S

WRITTEN BY

ROBERT K. ZIMMERMAN

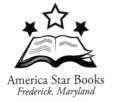

America Star Books
Frederick, Maryland

Second printing

America Star Books has allowed this work to remain exactly as the author intended, verbatim, without editorial input.

This publication contains the opinions and ideas of its author. Author intends to offer information of a general nature. Any reliance on the information herein is at the reader's own discretion.

The author and publisher specifically disclaim all responsibility for any liability, loss, or right, personal or otherwise, which is incurred as a consequence, directly or indirectly, of the use and application of any contents of this book. They further make no representations or warranties with respect to the accuracy or completeness of the contents of this work and specifically disclaim all warranties including without limitation any implied warranty of fitness for a particular purpose. Any recommendations are made without any guarantee on the part of the author or the publisher.

Paperback 9781635089073
Softcover 9781681762333
eBook 9781635089059
PUBLISHED BY AMERICA STAR BOOKS, LLLP
www.americastarbooks.pub
Frederick, Maryland

DEDICATION

This book is dedicated to my family. They have lived with me and thus with Parkinson's disease for the last twenty-six years. When I was diagnosed, Greg was twelve-years-old; Geoff, ten; Mark, eight; Matt, seven; Sarah, four; and Mary, two. Along with my wife Judy, they have been supportive, solicitous, and most helpful during this whole time. Judy, especially, has been my care partner and as such has been with me every step of the way. She has been my care partner for twenty-six out of our forty years of marriage.

Acknowledgements

My deepest appreciation to my son Greg, my sister Joyce Ann Zimmerman, C.PP.S., and my wife Judy for their proofing and editing of the manuscript. Their suggested changes were right on and made for a much richer book. Greg is a professional writer, Joyce is an accomplished author, and Judy is a retired high school English teacher. They all brought a unique view to the final manuscript. I especially appreciated the chapter Judy wrote on the role of the care partner.

INTRODUCTION

Expertise is not something that comes easily (what does?). Over the course of many years, through a combination of book study and life experiences, experts gradually acquire the knowledge and experience necessary to master a field. I have unwillingly become an expert on Parkinson's disease (PD) because I, as well as my wife and six children, have lived with Parkinson's for twenty-six years. This book is the story of our lives with Parkinson's.

People ask me all the time if I would be willing to talk to someone they know or love who has been diagnosed with the disease. I am always happy to do so and, as in those conversations, it's always important to start with a few basics. Dr. James Parkinson first described the disease in an English medical journal in 1817. He called it the "palsy disease," primarily because the most common manifestation is tremors.

So what exactly is Parkinson's disease? PD is a debilitating condition that affects the brain, specifically the movement center of the brain. There are cells in the brain called neurons which produce a chemical called dopamine. In the brain of a person with PD, for some unknown reason, these cells are dying. As the disease progresses the amount of dopamine decreases, leaving a person unable to control his or her movements. Most people know that when a person's hands shake, they have PD. There are, however, other symptoms that plague a person with PD. Muscle rigidity, slowness of movement, gait problems including balance (I lose my balance and fall on the average about once a month; others have told me I am unbalanced all the time) and coordination. Other related symptoms may include depression, fatigue, sleep disorders, dementia, and last, but certainly not least, constipation. All of these symptoms can vary from person to person.

Even today, the cause of the disease is unknown, although there are many theories. I have been asked if I drank well water when I was a child (well water with sulfur smelled and tasted like rotten eggs—yuck!) or lived on a farm, neither of which is true. There was a study done in Europe in the late 1990s that identified a number of families that showed more than one instance of Parkinson's disease among their members. There is small body of evidence that PD is a hereditary disease with Parkinson's disease showing up in more than one family member, thus lending credence to the theory that Parkinson's is hereditary. In my case, I am the only one in my immediate or extended family who has it. The more we learn about it, seemingly, the more we discover all that we don't know.

Parkinson's disease strikes both men and women (it's an equal opportunity disease!) and usually older people (fifty-five and up), although it is not uncommon for people in their thirties—actor Michael J. Fox is one well-known example—to have PD. It is a very difficult disease to diagnose because there is no blood test or x-ray that will give the neurologist a definitive answer. It must be clinically diagnosed which means the doctor must observe the person's movements. The neurologist should be an expert in the field of PD or, at the very least, a movement specialist. In my case, the fifth doctor I saw diagnosed my PD. He was a Parkinson's expert who worked at the PD clinic at the state university medical center. It is a difficult disease to diagnose and many people have told me that it took them up to year of chasing doctors before a definitive diagnosis was made. How prevalent is Parkinson's disease? These are only estimates, but there are about seven million people worldwide and more than one million in the United States with PD. Around 60,000 Americans will be

diagnosed each year. Incidence of PD increases w
the person (approximately four percent are diagnos
age fifty).

How does a doctor treat PD? Because there is no cure yet,
a doctor will treat the symptoms. The first line of attack is
a drug called "Levodopa." There are many other drugs that
work in concert (although I have never heard any music!)
with Levodopa. There is also a myriad of drugs that treat other
symptoms. At one point my shelf in the bathroom looked like
a pharmacy. My doctor told me early on in my disease that the
exercise I engaged in daily was just as good as the pills he was
prescribing for me.

An alternative treatment is a surgery called deep brain
stimulation (DBS). This surgery is good for only a small
number of people who fit a very strict set of criteria. I am one
of the fortunate people who have had the surgery and it has
allowed me to continue to be very active.

Can people die from Parkinson's disease? PD is a progressive
and debilitating disease that eventually robs people of their
ability to engage in a quality lifestyle. It, however, will not
cause their death directly. Usually heart attack, stroke, cancer,
pneumonia, kidney or liver failure, etc. will be the culprit. What
is interesting to me is that the course of the disease is never the
same for any two people. For some PD progresses very slowly
and for others it becomes quite debilitating in a short time.
For example, in as little as five years some people are unable
to function. In my case, the symptoms have progressed very
slowly.

But no matter the prognosis, a PD diagnosis can be a
bewildering, frightening time for the patient and his or her
family. My goal for this book is for others who read it benefit

from my years of reading, research, and simply living with this disease. By sharing my experiences, what I have learned and how I've coped with this disease, I'm hopeful that others with PD can learn to better cope with their own challenges with PD. This book is not meant to be a medical treatise, but rather a balanced look at one person's struggles and successes over the course of over a quarter of a century of life with this dreaded disease. Furthermore, the book is about my experiences with different doctors, different medications, and different reactions to the treatments. The book covers the deep brain stimulation (DBS) surgery I had with the resulting changes in my life. But mostly this book is about my family's journey of complete denial to eventual acceptance of PD.

The first chapter begins with the story of how I was diagnosed with PD and the various stages and issues I faced. I will also include some tips or things I learned early on that have really helped me cope through the years. The next chapter will deal with the early years of my living with PD and things I learned that helped me cope with the disease. Chapter 3 covers the events that led up to my decision to undergo deep brain stimulation (DBS) surgery. Chapter 4 describes the DBS surgery itself as well as the aftermath. The next chapter talks about my life after surgery. Chapter 6 covers my second surgery and life after it. Chapter 7 is written by my wife Judy and describes the importance of the care partner. I know I wouldn't be writing this book without her care and concern. Chapter 8 is the conclusion and gives some final thoughts. I hope that you enjoy reading this book as much as I enjoyed writing it!

CHAPTER 1
DIAGNOSIS

On December 19, 1988, I got a "pretty sure" diagnosis of Parkinson's disease. Approximately a year before I began to experience almost unnoticeable shaking in my right hand. I would only notice it when I was sitting still, not doing anything. As the year wore on, my right leg would drag so it looked like I was limping. I paid no attention to these symptoms because of my busy schedule. I thought the shaky hand was a result of stress due to my mother's terminal lung cancer. I had been driving forty miles round trip to my parents' home a couple times a week to help take care of her and make sure she was getting everything she needed. My dad was her primary caregiver but, when faced with the complexities of taking care of his sick wife, he would become very befuddled. When Mom died in August of 1988, I thought the shakes would go away. By the middle of September not only had they not gone away, but they were a little more pronounced. When my wife Judy convinced me to go see our family doctor, I made an appointment with my primary care physician, Dr. B, at the end of September. At this point I was feeling that we weren't going to find out anything and this was much ado about nothing. After all, I had just turned forty two. I exercised at the local YMCA, swimming laps almost every day for at least half-an-hour. I was otherwise in perfect health.

After Dr. B examined me, he did not want to speculate about a diagnosis. First he wanted to rule out any muscle or reflex problems. He made an appointment with a physiatrist, Dr. H. After sticking me with needles (I felt as though I was in a Chinese torture chamber) that were hooked up to a computer, Dr. H said my reflexes and muscles were all working just fine. Next, Dr. B made an appointment for me with Dr. S, a neurosurgeon. He ordered an MRI on my head. Dr. S concluded the results showed nothing out of the ordinary. At least I had empirical evidence that I did have a brain (humor is great medicine for those with PD). During this exam, my right leg showed slight tremors. Dr. S saw the tremor, but he also said he couldn't say what it was or what was causing it. He made an appointment for me with a movement specialist, Dr. M at The Ohio State University Medical Center. At this point I had been seen by our family doctor, Dr. B; a physiatrist, Dr. H; a neurosurgeon, Dr. S; and had an appointment (scheduled for December 19th, 1988) with a movement specialist, Dr. M.

After returning home from the appointment with Dr. S, my wife and I began a quest for information. We read about muscular dystrophy, multiple sclerosis, nervous disorders, and many other conditions but we did not consider Parkinson's disease. PD never came up in our research or our discussions prior to the appointment with Dr. M. I was feeling that this whole thing was just going to go away by itself and that I didn't really have any of these conditions we had read about. I really didn't think I had anything to worry about. It was clearly a case of denial.

My appointment with Dr. M was scheduled for 8:30 AM, so I had to leave Sidney, Ohio, early (about 7:00 AM) to drive the hour-and-a-half to The Ohio State University Medical Center. He walked into the examining room and began with the usual questions. After observing me he said, "You have Parkinson's disease." He then handed me a prescription for Sinemet which is the first medication that doctors usually prescribe for PD. At that time it was also the most effective medicine that could be taken. He then asked me if I had any questions. I began asking questions like what causes it, what can I expect in the future, what are these pills suppose to do, will I have to take this medicine for the rest of my life? He looked at me and said, "You had no clue that your condition was PD, did you?" I nodded. He very patiently answered all of my questions and even went a step further. He called The Ohio State's Movement Disorder Center's neurologist, Dr. P and made an appointment for me that same day at noon. I was sure that Dr. P was giving up his lunch hour so he could meet with me. I will always remember the kindness of the two OSU Medical Center doctors. I think they both understood my feelings of fear, confusion, anger, and frustration upon finding out the diagnosis of PD.

The thing I remember most about that morning was my phone call home to tell Judy, my wife, that PD was the probable culprit of my shakes. One of the first things I remember telling her was relief that it was not multiple sclerosis. Her reaction was similar to mine: total disbelief. People my age don't get PD! Why hadn't we considered PD as a possibility when we were researching? She felt awful that she wasn't with me for these two appointments, but we had six children twelve-years-old and under to take care of. I assured her that things would work out fine. I think I was trying to convince myself.

Dr. P was amazing. He spent a considerable amount of time examining me, observing my movements, and doing what I later learned were the standard neurological tests for people with PD. Then I began asking the questions I had been thinking of all morning. He answered each one very patiently. For example, he answered my first question about cause by saying there is no known cause, but the lack of the neurotransmitter, dopamine, in the brain was what was causing the symptoms. I asked him what the future holds. How long will I be able to work? He said the course of the disease is different for each of his patients. He certainly couldn't predict the future but, being young, I was in good physical shape because I exercised regularly, did not smoke, and ate healthy meals. He said I should be able to work for quite a few years. He asked me what I did for a living. I told him that I was superintendent of the Shelby County Board of Mental Retardation and Developmental Disabilities. He indicated that position was better for me than if I were, for example, engaged in manual labor or were a surgeon. I wondered if I should tell my board members. Some people tell the whole world and others try to hide the condition as long as they can.

Dr. P said he wanted to do two things just to confirm what he suspected. First, I was to have some blood drawn to rule out Huntington's disease, which is a very rare disease that manifests itself with slight tremors. Second, and more importantly, he told me to take the medicine (Sinemet) that Dr. M had prescribed to see if it had any effect on the symptoms. If the medicine did help the symptoms, then we would know for sure that it was Parkinson's disease. So, the day after I came home from Columbus, I had the blood test and passed that. It was not Huntington's disease. I began taking the Sinemet the next day. Dr. P suggested I start with one Sinemet per day for the next two days, then two pills per day, and three pills a day after two more days. The results were quite remarkable. The tremors stopped altogether and the stiff leg loosened up considerably. Dr. P had told me that muscle rigidity was one of the standard symptoms of Parkinson's disease. When I called his office with these results, he wanted to see me again on January 23, 1989. I was still in a state of disbelief or, more accurately, in a state of denial.

On the way home after that first appointment in Columbus on December 19, I decided I was going to tell people about my newly diagnosed disease. Telling people was the first baby step towards acceptance. When the next time the County Board of MR/DD (the board I worked for) met in mid-January, I told them as much as I knew at that point about my PD. They were totally supportive, although they asked how long I would be able to work. I gave them the same answer Dr. P had given me. The course of the disease is unknown because it is different for each person. I told the board that if my performance on the job lagged in any way I would be happy to step aside. They were more than satisfied with that explanation.

My wife Judy and I together decided that I would tell our children. We had been blessed with six ranging in age from two to twelve at the time of my diagnosis. They knew I'd had a number of doctor appointments over the last several months and they knew I had something wrong with me, but they had no clue what it was. Judy and I decided I would talk to each kid alone to explain PD on his or her level. Trying to explain it to a two-year-old was a bit challenging. They asked some very astute questions. One of their questions was whether I'd have to use a wheelchair some day? Another good question was, will you have to go to a nursing home when you get older? I had to answer them truthfully that I really didn't know. One asked me, why can't you just be cured? I told them that we can always hope. I told my five-year-old daughter that I was going to work very hard so that I could walk down the aisle with her at her wedding. This little encounter brought a tear to my eye.

Parkinson's is a chronic and progressive disease. I had read that keeping track of appointments, questions, and medication changes was important. So I started a notebook with all this information. That was such good advice because as the years flew by, there were changes in doctors, medicine changes, and new information about the disease. I was able to answer questions about past treatments and medication changes that I certainly would not have remembered. I also kept a folder with all the information, newsletters, etc. that I collected from day one. I have an amazing array of information by now.

Keeping notes also allowed me to feel that I was in charge of my disease. One strategy I also employed was that before an appointment, I would write in the notebook any questions Judy or I wanted to ask the doctor. I would then write the answers in the notebook after we asked the question. The only problem with this technique is that now it is hard for me to read my own handwriting.

Prior to the appointment on January 23, 1989, we (I am saying "we" at this point because from the beginning, Judy was my care partner, my morale booster, and my cheerleader) wrote a number of questions. Dr. P was very patient and answered every one of them. Would it be better to hold off taking Sinemet until I really needed it later in the disease? I had read that after a period of time a patient would experience an "on-off" effect. This means that at the end of a dose of Sinemet the benefit of the medication wears off and the symptoms return until the next dose of medicine kicks in. I had also read that the longer a patient takes Sinemet, the less beneficial it becomes. Dr. P stated he had heard that also but in his experience there were no data to support that claim. He also said he was giving me a minimal dosage of medicine at this point (three 100mg tablets per day).

What kind of exercise program besides swimming should I be on? He said swimming was a perfect exercise. On more than one occasion he indicated that the swimming was probably doing as much good for me as the pills he was prescribing for me. At this point I asked him if I would have to take these pills for the rest of my life. He nodded his head, "yes." Initially, I think that was one of the most distressing aspects of finding out I had PD. I had always prided myself on being healthy and in good shape physically. I weighed the same as the day I graduated from high school (no, I was not a heavyweight at my high school graduation!). I never even took aspirin for headaches because I never had headaches (my dad used to say that was because there was nothing up there to hurt!). The idea of being on medication for the rest of my life really bothered me.

We had read that stress may have made the symptoms appear. Is this possible? Dr. P answered that we really have no clue yet as to the cause. He said there was a lot of research presently being conducted. If these efforts continue, the future looks bright for an eventual cure. On a scale of one to ten, I asked him where my symptoms fell (one being the least bothersome and ten being the most bothersome). He indicated that I was at a one. How soon will I get to ten? He said he didn't know the answer, but probably somewhere between five and twenty years. I am at twenty-six years now, and I am at about a two or three. As I have said, the progression of the disease is different for each patient.

We all want to know what the future holds for us and I was no different, so I asked him again how long he thought I would be able to work. Dr. P said again and very astutely that he could not predict as the disease progresses differently with each patient he sees. I then told him I didn't know if it was my imagination, but since the day of my diagnosis, I noticed that I was a little more tired than before. I also told him that I felt a little depressed. He said that was normal. He said that researchers in the field are not sure if depression is caused by the disease itself or people are depressed upon learning that they have a chronic disease. Dr. P seemed to think the depression was one of the symptoms of the disease itself. If the depression became debilitating, he said he would prescribe a mild anti-depressant. That decision, he said, would be up to me. My feeling was that I didn't want to take anything else unless I absolutely had to. He agreed. As far as being tired, he simply said I probably need to get a little more rest. That sounded okay to me.

Somewhere in the first couple of months after my diagnosis in December and the appointment at the end of January, I decided that I simply was not going to let this disease get me down. I remember telling people, "I refuse to let Parkinson's disease intimidate me." Of course, that was easy to say when the symptoms were minimal. But I did figure out that besides exercise, a positive attitude was an extremely powerful antidote for the disease. As one example, after I had told my staff that I had Parkinson's, one of them had asked me if, when the weather outside was cold, were my tremors worse. My answer was, "Not if I stay warm." Another example of a positive attitude (and humor) was during a breakfast meeting, the person next to me was pouring herself a glass of orange juice. She read on the carton to shake and pour. I leaned over and said, "I bet I am the only person in this meeting who can do that at the same time." Making light of symptoms is always indicative of a positive attitude. So, very early on in the course of my disease, I had learned four vital things:
1. KEEP A POSITIVE ATTITUDE.
2. Get plenty of rest.
3. Get plenty of exercise.
4. Keep a notebook with all the information I gather.

The next question concerned diet. I wanted to know if there were any dietary restrictions or foods that would either help or hinder the symptoms. Dr. P didn't know of any and suggested I eat a normal, healthy diet. I told him that I read that vitamin E was good to take because it helped the body eliminate free radicals (cells floating inside the body that can cause disease). He said there was a large study being conducted nationwide, called the Data Top Study, which was investigating the effect of vitamin E on PD. Dr. P said it couldn't hurt and might have some positive effect, so he suggested I take 400 to 800 units per day. I have heard that other doctors have said that taking mega doses of any vitamin is wasting money. Or better put, "you eat 'em and excrete 'em." I took 800 units per day for years while the study was being conducted. The results of the study were inconclusive so I quit taking them. One more pill bottle off the shelf.

Although my diet was already healthy and, therefore, not something that needed to be changed, there were a couple of things that did negatively influence the slight tremors on my right side. Sugar was one of the nasty culprits. If I ate a couple of glazed donuts, for example, about an hour later my right hand and leg would tremor a little more than usual (I wouldn't have made it as a cop!). I really was not a dessert freak, but it was hard to give up the donuts. The other culprit I found was caffeine. It seemed to exacerbate the symptoms. I used to nurse a single cup of coffee all morning so that wasn't hard to give up, but Pepsi was another story. We ended that problem by simply never having pop with caffeine in the house anymore.

As with the first appointment, the appointment on January 23 went very well. Dr. P was again very patient with me. He suggested I come back in three months. I remember specifically asking him if he would continue to see me or would he transfer my care to someone else. His answer was, "It would be an honor to be your neurologist." As busy as he was with his teaching at The Ohio State University Medical Center, his research in the field of PD, and the clinic (The Madden Center of Excellence in Parkinson's disease at The Ohio State University), I felt he was always giving me his best. I was totally comfortable with him and the quality of the care I was receiving. He also made me feel that I was in control since it was my body and my disease. He always suggested things by saying a particular medicine or whatever is something he would recommend, rather than saying I have to take this or do that. And so I learned early on how important it is to be 100 percent comfortable with my doctor.

I felt very fortunate to have stumbled (literally) into Dr. P and the movement disorder clinic at The Ohio State University. But it is important to remember that the doctor is only as good as the information provided to him. He has to rely on the symptoms or conditions his patient shares with him in order to treat the patient effectively and efficiently. This is why it is critical to keep notebooks with all of our questions and answers; any changes since our last appointment; and copies of blood tests, x-ray reports, and other pertinent information.

After my December appointment (my initial diagnosis), I felt really down and in denial. By the end of the January appointment, I recognized a confidence in Dr. P that allowed me to feel that I was going to beat this disease or, at the very least, I was not going to let it keep me from doing what I wanted to do. I did have to make one concession, though; I told Judy I wouldn't go skydiving any longer. I had made three jumps before we were married, but none since.

I began to follow the regimen my doctor and I had worked out together. It makes no sense to me to go to a doctor and then not follow the treatment plan he or she prescribes. Deciding to have a positive attitude (gee, where have I said that before?) is the first step in the process of accepting the fact that one has a life-long disease.

Telling people up front that I have PD also helps me to cope with the effects of the disease. In my job I did a lot of public speaking. I would always start with telling the audience, "If I slur a word or can't seem to find the right word or you see my hand shake a little, it's not because I had something in my orange juice this morning. It is because I have P disease. Now that you know that, you won't sit wonder what's wrong with this guy. You will comfortable and so will I. Besides, now I can be nervous and you won't know the difference." I have had many people tell me they appreciated that little introduction.

During the time between the December diagnosis and the January appointment, Judy and I did a lot of research on PD. We found there were other symptoms that I did not show, but they could eventually present themselves. My PD began on my right side, but my symptoms were just the tremors and muscle rigidity. Also, my handwriting got very small and became almost illegible. Freezing, shuffling the feet, and balance are problems that many people with PD have. Freezing occurs when a person with PD's body literally stops motion. For example, a patient is walking or shuffling and all of sudden stops and can't move his or her feet any longer. Many people with PD have problems with balance. They are constantly falling down. I was very fortunate not to have been unbalanced (although some would dispute that fact!). Another common symptom of PD is bradykinesia. This symptom could be likened to someone trying to swim in a pool filled with molasses. Because the muscles are extremely rigid, movement is very slow. Luckily, I haven't experienced that symptom either.

It has been twenty-six years since I was diagnosed with PD, and I remember that day as if it were yesterday. I was extremely fortunate to have had doctors who kept digging until we came up with a diagnosis. I was also very lucky to have been referred to the movement center and, specifically, Dr. P. This chapter covered the issues and events that led up to my December 19, 1988, diagnosis as well as the information gathered at my January 23, 1989, appointment.

Chapter 2 will cover my life with PD for the next several years with explanations of how the disease progressed. I will also describe other things I learned that have helped me cope with PD. This period was marked by the slow progression of my disease, the changes in medications, and the various research projects in which the Madden Center for PD at Ohio State was involved.

CHAPTER 2
LIFE WITH PD

Sinemet was the best medication at that time for the beginning stages of the disease. I started out by taking three 25/100 mg tablets per day. Sinemet is a combination of Carbidopa (the 25mg) and Levodopa (the 100mg). When Levodopa was first introduced, it was given by itself with nausea and upset stomach being a widespread side effect. When combined with Carbidoba, patients tolerated the Levodopa much better.

With the three tablets per day that Dr. P prescribed for me, I had no nausea or upset stomach at all (it must be due to my cast iron German stomach!). Dr. P wanted to see me every three months, so my next appointment was in May, 1989.

Because he also taught at The Ohio State University and conducted research, Dr. P had clinic (saw patients) usually only on Mondays and Fridays. Since I was driving an hour and a half to Columbus, he said that if I could combine the visit to Ohio State with a trip to Columbus connected with my job on another day, he would be glad to accommodate me. Since I went to Columbus about once a month for my job, I took advantage of his generosity on a number of occasions.

Other than taking the three pills a day, my life didn't change much from pre-PD. I went to work every day, had a nice family dinner every night, played with the kids, and read bedtime stories (*Where the Wild Things Are* by Maurice Sendak was one of my favorites.) I became very busy after my election to the local hospital's board of trustees. There was usually one evening meeting per month and many committee meetings at 7:00 in the morning before work. That was a nine-year commitment and I served as chairman of the board for two of those years.

I flew along the next several years on auto-pilot without a great amount of difficulty. I constantly tried to sort out my feelings about having PD, but since my symptoms were still pretty mild, I kept doing what I had always done.

Then it hit me. A book I had read several years before, *On Death and Dying* by Elizabeth Kubler-Ross, outlined the steps of grieving that most people go through when they lose someone close to them. These five stages include denial, anger, bargaining, depression and finally full acceptance. I was going through a similar process, but didn't recognize it. It wasn't the death of someone close to me, but rather I was grieving the loss of my good health and the fact that PD would simply (or not so simply) keep getting more and more debilitating. There are no timelines for any of the stages of dealing with grief and no clear cut ending point for one stage and the beginning of the next. I have a pretty laid back type of a personality, so I can't remember ever being angry (besides, I was never sure with whom or at what to be angry). I was frustrated at times that I was not the healthy person I had always prided myself in being. I have definitely gone through times of depression; however, several doctors told me that people become depressed over the fact that they have PD, but also because of the imbalances of the chemistry of the brain. Whatever the cause of the depression, it is real and can be very debilitating in itself.

Of course, there are different levels of depression in any given patient. For me some of the signs were that I felt draggy all day and just didn't feel like doing anything. I wanted to stay curled up in my nice warm little bed until late in the morning, especially on weekends. This lasted only a month or so before my conscience in the form of my wife Judy intervened. She suggested I talk to the neurologist during my next visit. After discussing what was happening, the doctor started me on a mild anti-depressant (Wellbutrin). Sure enough, it worked amazingly well.

The last stage in this progression of grieving steps is acceptance. It seems that most people reach this plateau in about a year's time (although, I am not sure if I have ever fully accepted the disease). I go through periods when I don't think about it very much, and other times I dwell on it *ad nauseam*. Usually right before I had a doctor's appointment, I would flip between denial (why me?) and being upset at having to drive all the way to Columbus (which is about ninety miles) for Dr. P to tell me that I was doing just great; I should keep doing what I was doing. On the way home from these visits, I would usually say to myself, "Self, you will just have to play the hand that was dealt you." Also, I would remind myself that rule number one is *keep a positive attitude*. Within the last year or so I have thought about my PD as a blessing. I have had so many positive experiences and met so many wonderful people who have influenced my life. But even with these positive thoughts, the "why me?" question still nags me. And I suppose it will into the future. This is simply being human.

Approximately five years after getting a positive diagnosis, the symptoms began to appear a bit more noticeably. I noticed that the dosage of Sinemet that I was taking began "wearing off" about half-an-hour before I was due for the next dose. The new dose took half-an-hour to "kick in," so I was on my own for about an hour. On the next trip to the clinic at The Ohio State University, Dr. P began to adjust my medications, always very conservatively. One of the first ones he tried me on was Eldypril, which was intended to even out the "on-off" effect. It was also said to be neuroprotective (protecting the little bit of dopamine I still had), although studies still needed to verify that.

Dr. P then asked me if I was interested in participating in any clinical trials. One that he had in mind for me was the use of a patch to deliver the drug Eldypril through the skin. He explained that this was a double blind study (is this where the term "the blind leading the blind" came from?). This means that the two groups (experimental [often referred to as guinea pig] and control) did not know whether they were receiving a placebo or the real deal. The way this study was set up, the principal investigator also did not know. After agreeing to be in the study, Dr. P gave me the informed consent form which was very detailed.

The study started with a box of patches and instructions on how to fill out the daily data sheet. This log sheet contained information on the "on-off" time. Very quickly, in a matter of two or three days, I knew I was in the group receiving the real thing. My "on-off" periods became virtually nonexistent. I wondered if I really had PD. But, alas, all good things must come to an end. The study stopped because it was determined there was not going to be a big enough market (translation: people weren't going to make gazillion dollars from it). And so the study was stopped in the middle. Within a week or so my "on-off" symptoms returned. I was very frustrated, to say the least.

This was my first foray into the world of clinical trials. Why would I want to do something like that? I'm often asked. My response is always the same, "If it would help me or someone else in the future, that would be wonderful." Less than one percent of people with PD have participated in a clinical trial. The Parkinson's Disease Foundation (a national organization located in New York City) is working hard to change this level of participation. They have trained over 400 people from all over the country who operate as research advocates. The function of the advocate is to make people aware of clinical trials that are going on in the centers for PD. They are also working to bring awareness of PD to their communities. I attended an advocacy training session in October of 2010; it was an amazing experience.

There were about thirty people in attendance with varying stages of the disease. I felt right at home with all of these people with PD who were willing to spend their time working with people in their communities to bring awareness of Parkinson's, and to let folks know how they could become involved in clinical trials. But I am getting ahead of myself; more about this topic later.

During this period, my wife Judy and I kept reading to learn as much about the disease as possible. A couple things stand out. Choosing to have a positive attitude was the most important lesson we learned (haven't I mentioned that already?). I think part of having a positive attitude is telling other people that I have the disease and not just work associates and other acquaintances. I have heard of many people who try to hide their disease as long as possible because they are embarrassed by it. Other people I have heard about have decided to just stay home and never go out for fear of being stared at or ridiculed. I have not found this to be the case. I find most people are very helpful especially if they know what I have. I remember a situation that occurred at a major league baseball game a couple of years ago. It was towards the end of the game (which, by the way my team lost) when all of a sudden I had to go to the bathroom. I got up and squeezed by the people in my row and as I started up the steep steps, I stumbled over the first step. Quickly righting myself, I scurried up a couple more steps before I stumbled again, this time falling on the person sitting next to the aisle. Embarrassed, I just said, "Sorry," and went on. By this time the attendant was at my side and helped me up the rest of the way. It dawned on me that the people watching me for sure thought I had had too many beers. I turned to the attendant and said, "I have Parkinson's disease." She simply asked me if I was ok. On the way back to my seat a little later, I announced in a rather loud voice, "I'm sorry I fell on some of you people but I have Parkinson's, not too much beer." There were a number of smiles as I found my way back to my seat.

Judy and my continuing research also covered the necessity and value of regular exercise. I cannot emphasize enough how important getting regular exercise is. My form of exercise was swimming laps at the local YMCA. I had been swimming at the Y before my diagnosis, and so it was natural to continue. My normal routine was to swim a half mile which usually took me about thirty-five minutes. I did this during my lunch hour so it wouldn't disturb my time with the family. Making a game of it, I kept track of the number of miles I swam, going about 1,500 miles during the ten years I swam. Approximately eight of those years were after my diagnosis. I continued swimming until I began to lose the strength in my legs from the lack of coordination and muscle rigidity. I think I was swallowing more water than I was displacing, because I would go back to work and spend most of the rest of the afternoon in the bathroom. Eventually I had to give up swimming.

So, the next best thing to do was simply to find another form of exercise. The Y was very helpful by designing a program of weight lifting and aerobic exercise. I enjoyed that because there were lots of different machines such as treadmills, stationary bikes, stair masters, and even a rowing machine. For the weight training there was a full nautilus setup which made it very easy to get a good workout in about half-an-hour.

There was always a TV in the exercise room so it was not so boring.

When I was unable to lift anymore, I began a routine of walking. In the winter I walked on our treadmill in the basement of our home or I used the elliptical machine. During the rest of the year I walked our neighborhood sidewalks at least thirty minutes a day. I tried to do two miles in that thirty-minute workout and when I felt good I would stretch that to forty- to forty-five minutes. It was hard to do that every day with our busy schedules, but I always walked a minimum of three days a week.

There are other kinds of programs that people with PD can enjoy as well. Yoga and Tai Chi come to mind. I tried Tai Chi for about a month, and I was a dismal failure at it. I could breathe the right way and I could do some of the steps the right way, but when I tried to put them together, it simply did not work. I would either fall over or turn blue. So I went back to walking (I did not attempt to chew bubble gum while walking, though!).

Another area Judy and I researched was diet. We found out that certain foods were deadly for my symptoms and others were great. For example, while I was never a big coffee drinker I did enjoy a one cup in the morning at work. There was a little warmer on my desk, so I would nurse a cup all morning long. I usually didn't have any at home on weekends. It took me a year or so to figure out that the caffeine in the coffee added to my tremors. So I cut out all foods with caffeine, and was a bit calmer. A deadly combination I figured out was donuts or sweet rolls with coffee in the morning. I did not eat donuts that often but when I did, I experienced big time tremors about an hour or so after ingesting with great gusto a couple of donuts.

The logical thing was to cut out all processed sugar from my diet as much as possible.

I also learned that protein tended to interfere with the Parkinson's medication, making it less effective. I followed the suggestion Dr. P gave me and tried to eat foods with protein at night. Peanuts became a favorite snack at bed time. I was taking Sinemet four times a day and was told that they would be more effective if I took them about thirty- to forty-five minutes before eating. If that weren't possible, taking them about two hours after eating aided in their effectiveness.

Smoking is another no-no for lots of reasons. I had smoked in college and for a year for so after college, but have been smoke free for about forty years now. Giving up smoking was not difficult at all.

Drinking alcohol was another story. I used to enjoy a glass of wine with dinner every once in a while, and a beer with pizza. When I read that alcohol was possibly connected to the depression that came along with Parkinson's, I was a little frustrated and depressed. On this one I cheated once in a while because I was going to be depressed anyway. But other than a few indulgences on major holidays, I am pretty good about abstaining from beer and wine.

To summarize, then, the things I learned in the first year after my diagnosis:
1. Have a POSITIVE ATTITUDE.
2. Keep a notebook which contains all of the questions and answers, what was discussed at an appointment, and any test results or reports.
3. Exercise regularly. If one needs help with coming up with a routine, there are many programs specifically geared towards people with Parkinson's (the BIG program is

geared to slowing down the progression of the disease; the LOUD program is excellent for keeping one's voice level understandable).

4. Make the most out of appointments by coming prepared with questions and, after the appointment, do what the doctor suggests. This way one is a participant in one's own care.
5. Decide to have a positive attitude.
6. Develop a sense of humor about Parkinson's.
7. Cut out caffeine and alcohol from the diet and eat healthy meals and snacks. Try to eat protein only at the evening meal.
8. Have a positive attitude.
9. Try to take Sinemet about a half hour to forty-five minutes before eating a meal.
10. You guessed it: Have a positive attitude.

Nothing much changed in the first five years after my diagnosis. Dr. P had said that many people begin to really have difficulties right around the five-year mark. I was still working and carrying out my full schedule. The board I worked for was still very understanding as well as supportive. In the fall of 1993 I began to notice very slight tremors on my left side. I probably wouldn't have noticed it except I had experienced the same thing on my right side. Remember, I said it was a year from the time I notice the symptoms on my right side until I went to the doctor.

Between my fifth-year and tenth-year anniversary (1998), I began to notice that the "on" and "off" effect was much more prevalent. Since my symptoms were still pretty mild (I guess they weren't pretty—just mild), it didn't really bother me all that much. Dr. P adjusted my medication a little bit and we were off to the races again. He always told me he tended to under-medicate me so we would save the heavier duty bullets for when the disease really kicked in. Fortunately, this didn't happen until much later in the disease progression.

At about this ten-year mark I received a letter from The Ohio State Medical Center saying that Dr. P was retiring but would be at the clinic on a minimal schedule. The letter also introduced Dr. H as his full time replacement. I felt sad that I would no longer be able to work with Dr. P, but Dr. H was a terrific replacement. She carried on his tradition. The most important aspect of this change for me was that Dr. H also made me feel part of the decision-making team. My input counted and she listened supportively. But she was only at the movement clinic three years when she took another position. I was very sorry to see her go as well. Dr. K, another neurologist and my third PD doctor, took over and I was very fortunate that she trained in the Dr. P system.

The only problem was that Dr. K only stayed until the fall of 2002. We got another letter from The Ohio State University Medical Center telling us that Dr. K took another position. This time there was no replacement for her. So, I had my choice of waiting six months to make an appointment with a Dr. T who was part time at the clinic, or I could see one of the nurses. At that time my three month check up was due, and if I had to wait six more months after that I felt that would be a problem. Needless to say, I was a bit perturbed; doctors were supposed to stay in one spot for their whole career, especially the good ones, right?

The day after we got the news that Dr. K was moving on, a flyer arrived in the mail from the Cleveland Clinic announcing a new program for people with Parkinson's. What a great bit of serendipity! The program consisted of a multi-disciplinary evaluation, which consisted of a physical therapist (PT), an occupational therapist (OT), a speech therapist, an activities therapist, a physician's assistant, and a neurologist. I had never had a complete work up like this, so I was pretty excited. We made an appointment for a couple of weeks from that initial phone call. They told us it would last about four hours or more. The only problem we could foresee was that Cleveland was about four hours from our home, much farther than Columbus. We are very fortunate that Judy's brother lives about ten minutes from the Cleveland Clinic. He told us we were welcome to stay at his house any time we needed to be in Cleveland. We certainly took advantage of his generosity over the next several years, which leads us to the content of the next chapter. Chapter 3 includes the time from 2004 until the spring of 2006 and the events that led up to our decision to undergo deep brain surgery (DBS).

CHAPTER 3
DECIDING TO HAVE DBS SURGERY

The year 2004 turned out to be very eventful. In February of that year I was diagnosed with cancer in the form of non-Hodgkin's lymphoma. I said to myself, "Keep a positive attitude." The oncologist who treated my cancer was excellent. We started treatment with a trip to the hospital to get two bags of platelets because my level was at 6,000—a normal low is 150,000. I wasn't sure of what that meant until Dr. K, my new best friend and oncologist, said that platelets were vital to the blood being able to clot. I asked him that, if I cut myself shaving tomorrow morning, could I bleed to death. He indicated it would have to be a pretty deep cut, but essentially I had the right idea.

Then we started the chemo routine. I was to receive eight doses of the cocktail, a dose administered every three weeks. Everything was going smoothly until about half way through the treatments I then developed an upper respiratory infection. That little infection landed me in the hospital for about two weeks because the doctors couldn't figure out what was causing it. The doctors told me the infection was significant because my immune system was severely compromised due to the chemo treatments. The infection finally surrendered to treatment and I was able to go home with a pretty powerful anti-biotic and an oxygen machine.

During the second week in the hospital, Judy and I talked about the possibility of my retiring. We decided that it would be a very prudent move. I did not want to come back to a very demanding job, possibly screw it up, or become completely ineffective. The Shelby County Board of Mental Retardation and Developmental Disabilities agreed and accepted my retirement request. I had thirty-three years in the state public retirement system, was fifty-eight years old, and could retire with full benefits. While I was sick in the hospital, I arranged for a friend of mine (A) who held her superintendent's certificate to come to Shelby County as an interim superintendent. She was more than glad to do this and immediately became interested in the job full time. I was relieved because what I had worked hard for would continue in A's capable hands. With all the paid time off I had accumulated, the Board of MR/DD made the effective date of my retirement December 31, 2004. I was grateful to the board for their acceptance of my request.

My last chemo treatment was August 1, 2004. After a PET scan towards the end of the month, I was declared officially in remission on September 1, 2004. The chemo treatments left me tired and draggy for the next four months, making us very glad that I had retired. In no way, shape, or form would I have been able to perform my job to the standard the board required of its superintendent.

But retirement seldom means doing nothing. On January 2, 2005, I volunteered to be the interim director for the Shelby County Libraries. I was on the board of trustees for the library system; the board wanted someone there to search for a new director. Also I was asked to keep the lid on the boiling pot until the new permanent person was in place. Our library system consists of the main library and five other smaller libraries sprinkled around the county. I worked about thirty hours a week, so it wasn't nearly as taxing as my superintendent job was. There was some stress, but fortunately not enough to affect my PD symptoms. I really enjoyed my time at the library and turned the reins over to the more-than-capable hands of S in June of 2005. She turned out to be a superb director and an excellent administrator. We felt very fortunate to have found someone as capable as S. So, I retired a second time after six months in the interim director's position.

In November of 2005 Judy and I traveled to Cleveland for the comprehensive evaluation. After being evaluated by the PT, OT, speech pathologist, and the activities therapist, I met with S, a nurse practitioner. She took down my medical history in great detail. Then she turned me over to Dr. G, a neurologist who specialized in Parkinson's disease and other related movement disorders. This doctor turned out to be a wonderful find. After Dr. G and S talked, Dr. G met with me. Dr. G first examined me and then said, "You would be a perfect candidate for deep brain stimulation (DBS) surgery." I must have looked dumfounded as I told her I had never heard of DBS. We spent over an hour going over the procedure, the treatment, and all it would entail. Her most interesting comment was explaining that how I feel in the morning right when my morning medications kick in is how I would feel all day long. I told her that I felt terrific and at those times I wondered if a really had the disease. She explained that in my case, with the DBS I would feel that good all day. Wow, did that ring my bell!

She further explained that the surgery would be performed by Dr. R, a neurosurgeon who had done more of these procedures than anyone else in the world. At that time she said there were only about 40,000 people in the whole wide world who had had the surgery done. She explained that the procedure was approved by the Federal Drug Administration (FDA), which means that it was no longer considered to be an experimental treatment for people with PD. I asked her what the long term prognosis was and how long ago the first couple procedures were done. She explained that they have been following a patient who had it done experimentally ten years before. She said he was still doing very well.

The procedure entailed drilling two dime-sized holes into my cranial bone. Dr. R would then fish two wires into my brain until he found the small movement center in the brain. The exciting part of this operation was that I would be awake and participating in the procedure. Another positive aspect of this surgery is if a cure for PD is ever found, the surgeon could remove the system without any harm.

The process for determining whether I was a candidate for the surgery was a complicated one. A team of doctors and therapists would each do their evaluations and then decide whether I was a candidate or not. The first evaluation was a complete neuropsychological exam. The purpose of these exercises was to determine a baseline for areas such as short- and long-term memory, verbal skills, reading comprehension, etc. A baseline is simply an assessment of performance that can be compared to data collected after the surgery. After the surgery and the transmitters were programmed and functioning the way they were supposed to, the psychologists would give the same test to see if I had gained or lost any of the skills (I still maintain the tests were given to see if I was crazy enough to have the DBS procedure performed or not!). It is a long and demanding surgery.

After explaining all this information, Dr. G told us that we should think about it and then decide whether I wanted to be considered for the surgery. We were then supposed to call her with a decision by the end of December. Judy and I felt very optimistic with the exam and the information we picked up. We went into our "due diligence" mode and read everything we could about DBS. One of the things we found out was that there was a three percent chance of complications or side effects with the surgery. Some of those included paralysis, stroke, or even death, to name just a few. We ended up by deciding that three chances in one hundred for negative side effects were pretty long odds especially if the results were as good as they sounded. I asked Dr. G if she knew any patients who had the surgery and would be willing to answer my questions. She said it was a good idea. She gave me Mr. C's name and phone number.

Before we actually decided to request the opportunity to be a candidate I called Mr. C who had already had the DBS surgery and asked him his experience with the procedure. He was very generous with his time and he answered all my questions. This PD patient had had a complication of an infection which meant that he had to have the operation performed a second time. He felt so strongly about the benefits on one side that he chose to go through the surgery a second time. He also told me that if I decided to go through with the surgery, I should join his online support group called the "Live Wires." I thanked him for his honest experiences. He assured me that he wasn't giving me a recommendation, but only sharing his unique experiences. I really appreciated his whole approach.

Based on all the information we had gathered and the discussions with Mr. C, Judy and I decided it was definitely worth the effort. I called Dr. G to tell her we would like to be considered for the surgery. She said she would get back with me in a couple of weeks with the team's yea or nay to my being a candidate. Exactly two weeks later Dr. G called to inform me that they would like to consider me for the surgery. The first week in January, 2006, the Cleveland Clinic's Office of Neurological Restoration called with a schedule of appointments. The first was with Dr. G. I was to come in without taking my normal medications so they could observe me when I was "off" medicine. Then they told me to take my medicine and they would evaluate me again. This visit was meant to determine how severe my symptoms were both off and on the medication. They next asked me what three things I expected from the surgery. This question was asked of me throughout the rest of the process every time I had an appointment. My answer was consistent: the first expectation was better control over the tremors, the second was a lessoning of the muscle rigidity, and the third was an end to the dyskinesia (dyskinesia is the result of too much medication and is characterized by large random movements, especially of the arms). If the doses of medicine are reduced in order to control the dyskinesia, the other symptoms such as tremors, rigidity, and slowness of movement increase dramatically. At this point I had been diagnosed for some sixteen years, and the only thing I could think was that the disease was going to get worse. So, why shouldn't I try to get as many good years as I could? Judy really helped me put this into perspective when she said, "You will want to enjoy your grandchildren." I wanted to get on with the surgery as quickly as possible.

After going through the battery of neurological tests, neuropsychological tests, and the normal tests to determine if I could physically stand the stress of brain surgery, I was given a date for the surgery. Judy had to go through a psychology exam also. The surgery was to be performed on May 1, 2006, which also happened to be my oldest daughter Sarah's twenty-second birthday. She didn't sound real thrilled about spending her birthday in a hospital. I told her and the other kids that this was no big deal and that they didn't need to come. They all said brain surgery *was* a big deal and they wanted to be there. I have to say I was really pleased that all but two of our six children were able to be there to root their dad on.

After listening to the particulars of the surgery, I didn't feel apprehensive until the day before the trip to Cleveland. I wasn't really worried because the doctors had made me feel that this whole thing was pretty routine. They told me I would be awake for most of the surgery and what I should expect.

The next chapter deals with the surgery itself as well as the aftermath.

CHAPTER 4
DBS–THE ACTUAL SURGERY

I was scheduled to be admitted into the hospital on Sunday afternoon, April 30, 2006; I was told they were going to begin at 6:30 sharp the next morning. I slept really well that night which was surprising since I was anticipating the surgery. At exactly 6:30 AM the resident neurologist came into my room. He said he was there to put on a stereotactic headgear apparatus. The purpose was so I wouldn't move my head during surgery. The headgear, once in place, would be bolted to the operating table. The headgear was attached to my head with four screws, two in my forehead and two in the back of my head. They gave me a local anesthetic at each of the four sites where the screws were to be inserted. Oh, I almost forgot to mention that before they put this gear on, they completely shaved me bald (it was to be the most expensive haircut I ever got!). The screws were titanium and were actually put in with an ordinary screw driver. The doctor told me there would be no pain, only a little feeling of pressure when the screws went in. He was right. I really didn't feel anything other than a little push when he actually put the screws in.

Next was a wheelchair ride down to right outside of the waiting area for families, where my family was waiting to say goodbye or good luck or whatever else you say to people looking like I did. They looked at me like they were deer caught in a headlight. The kids were definitely freaked out by what I must have looked like with that halo on and a bald head. After all the standard "I love yous," I was wheeled down to the operating room where they literally bolted my head gear frame onto the table. Again, the tool they used looked like the average wrench from the local hardware store.

When I was wheeled into the operating room, I was completely amazed at the number of people in white lab jackets and scrubs. I remember thinking, "All these people are going to be working on me?" Everyone was extremely pleasant and explained things to me step by step. I was put to sleep first of all so they could drill two holes about the size of dimes in my skull. That gave the surgeons access to the part of the brain where they would put the probes. Then they woke me up and reassured me again the procedure would not hurt because there were no nerve endings in the brain. It seemed like it was forever before Dr. R came in and said the computer wasn't working right, but they had a backup they were going to bring in. I remember thinking that I hoped the backup was just as new and as up to date and as the one they were replacing. It seemed like a long time before Dr. R said they were ready to put in the probes. I didn't have any idea what time it was (they didn't have a clock on the ceiling).

The Cleveland Clinic had done an MRI and a CT scan in preparation for the procedure. The one was superimposed on top of the other so the surgeons could map the path they chose to put in the wires. I thought it was really cool; I could hear different noises as Dr. R fished the wire down to the subthalamus region of the brain. Dr. R said the noises were one of the ways they knew they were heading in the right direction (GPS systems apparently were of no help!). The probe had four leads which were then attached to the movement center of the brain (about the size of a dime again). Dr. C, another neurologist on the team, began to move my arm to test for rigidity and then they turned on the stimulator. I could immediately feel a relaxation of the whole right side of my body. At that point I wanted them to leave it on. But, alas, all good things come to an end and when they were sure they had the best lead—as I said there were four leads—they were ready to do the other side.

Dr. R asked me if I wanted to continue with doing the right side of my brain or come back another day since the left side of my brain had taken so long. I said it depended on how he felt, but I was ready to go for it (all I had to do was lie on the operating table with my head bolted down and smile once in a while). After doing the left side, Dr. R put me back to sleep to coil the wires under my scalp. These were the wires that would be fished down the side of my head and hooked to the transmitters which would be placed on either side of my upper chest just under the skin. This would be a second procedure to be done on an outpatient basis scheduled for a couple of weeks after the wires were put in.

When I woke up in the recovery room I found out that the operation lasted a little over twelve hours, but it didn't seem like that long to me. Judy thought it would never be over although the staff was really good about going out into the waiting area to tell Judy and the kids what was happening. The nurses had told me to bring my favorite CDs so they could play them while I was in the operating room. One of them was Credence Clearwater Revival's greatest hits, which was playing when I woke up at the beginning of the operation. I think they thought it was a little too jazzy, so they played something a little more soothing after that.

Dr. R came into the recovery room after I woke up Monday night to ask me how I was feeling. I was great; no pain whatsoever. As it turned out there was never any pain. Everyone's pain tolerance level is different. Dr. R did a CT scan after the operation to make sure everything was in order. He said the probes on the right side of my head which controls movement on the left side on my body had somehow coiled up and they did not think they could be turned on. He seemed genuinely concerned because he said that had never happened to him before (I said that made two of us; it had never happened to me before either!). We would wait until the left side was turned on to see if there was any crossover effect. Then we would decide what to do.

My whole head was wrapped in white gauze like a swami, although at that point I really didn't care what I looked like. I stayed in the recovery area overnight Monday night and was moved to a room on Tuesday morning. I felt great all day Tuesday. On Wednesday morning Dr. R said I could go home. I don't remember much of the trip home as I slept most of the four hours it took us to get back to Sidney.

What was really interesting was that by Friday of that week I felt really good. I took off the dressings on my head on Friday. My head looked like the stitching on a baseball. Although Dr. R prescribed pain pills, I never felt like I needed them from the time I got home on Wednesday. My PD symptoms were much better for about two weeks after the surgery. Dr. R said that was pretty typical because the wire probes in the movement center swelled the brain a tiny bit which resulted in the symptoms being better.

Two weeks after the surgery we went back to the Cleveland Clinic for the outpatient procedure to hook up the wires to the battery packs. That procedure was a piece of cake. We went home immediately after I woke up and could keep some food down. Again I was in no pain or even discomfort from the surgery.

The next step in the process was to turn on the stimulator and begin to program it. S, nurse practitioner and chief programmer, did the honors. This occurred two weeks after the battery packs were implanted. She said we would gradually kick up the juice over the next six weeks in order to get maximum benefit. After she reached the best settings I couldn't believe how good I felt. The tremors on the right side of my body were completely eliminated, as was the dyskinesia. My muscles seemed to loosen up also. This was all on the right side of my body, while the symptoms were still present on the left side of the body because that side wasn't hooked up yet. They couldn't turn it on due to the coiled wires. The doctors were hoping there would be some crossover effect that would aid the left side of the body. But by the autumn of 2006 it became apparent that the crossover effect hoped for was not going to happen. Both Dr. G and Dr. R recommended that we redo the surgery on the right side of my brain. So, the surgery was scheduled for January 10, 2007. Man was I pumped! After all, I had gone through this whole process once before. And both sides were then going to function in tandem again.

My experience with the second surgery was very similar to the first. I was in the operating room about eight hours instead of the twelve for the first surgery. All went well and I was allowed to go home on the third day after surgery. I went back in a couple of weeks for the stimulator to be turned on and programmed. It took about four sessions of programming to get it just right. This time Dr. R said the team hit the nail perfectly on the head (so to speak). Interestingly enough, the voltage used on the right side of the brain was exactly the same setting as the one on the left side (3. 6 volts).

As mentioned previously, we were very fortunate that Judy's brother Jim lives ten minutes or so from the Cleveland Clinic. He graciously provided lodging for us on every trip to the clinic. Otherwise, it would have been very costly to stay in hotels and eat our meals out. My bald head looked like the stitching on a baseball again. Our family physician Dr. B took out the stitches which saved us a return trip to Cleveland.

I was told that there were only about 40,000 people in the world who have had this surgery. So I was a member of a very exclusive club. Dr. R had performed more procedures than anyone else in the world. He was definitely considered the guru of deep brain stimulation surgery.

In the next Chapter I will talk about life after the surgery. Somehow, the local newspaper got the story and published a half-page article complete with a picture of Judy and me. That article generated a lot of interest in the procedure as evidenced by the number of phone calls I got asking me more details about my surgery. Some of these calls came as long as four years after the article appeared.

CHAPTER 5
LIFE AFTER SURGERY

Dr. R told me that the second surgery (1/10/07) went very well. He said he hit the right spot just perfectly with the wires; he was very happy with how it turned out. Of course if he was happy, then I was happy. As with the first surgery, the stimulator was turned on and programmed at the same voltage as the one on the other side (3.6 volts). Once it was turned on I can't say often enough about how good I felt. The two sides of my body were back in sync. The tremors were completely gone all day long. My muscles were much less rigid and my coordination seemed to be much better also. When I was asked at the beginning of the process what three things I hoped to accomplish with the surgery, I had said I wanted the tremors to be gone, the dyskinesia to be gone, and to have less muscle rigidity. As far as I was concerned at this point, Dr. R had hit a grand slam!

After programming the stimulator was finished, the next thing to attack was the medications I was taking prior to the surgeries. I don't remember all the "stuff" I was on, but I do remember that I took a 50mg tablet of Stelevo four times a day. Stelevo was a combination of three medicines: Carbidoba, Levodopa, and Entacopone. After the surgery I no longer felt the "on" and "off" phenomenon. I felt so good there were times when I would forget to take my medicine and I would not feel any different. Eventually I went down to three pills per day.

What was even more exciting was that I was scheduled for follow up visits only once every six months unless there was some kind of a problem with the system. About a year later Dr. G and S (my neurologist and my programmer) moved out of state to start a new movement disorders clinic. I had to decide whether to stay with the Cleveland Clinic and have a new neurologist or to move to a hospital somewhere else. Since my records were there already and because I was familiar with Dr. C, we decided to stay with the doctors in Cleveland. A trip to Cleveland every six months was not a major problem.

Shortly after I was programmed on both sides, the local newspaper wrote an article about my DBS surgery complete with a picture of Judy and me holding the little gizmo that turns the system on and off. I called it my "personal garage door opener." There were many phone calls from people with Parkinson's disease who wanted to know more about DBS and my experience with the surgery. As a result of those phone calls, Judy and I decided that a support group would be a good idea; at the time Sidney didn't have one. We arranged the first meeting at a room at the Sidney-Shelby County YMCA and put out the word through the newspaper and word of mouth when the first meeting was scheduled. We told people the group was for people with Parkinson's, people who had had DBS, people who were thinking about the surgery, and people with essential tremor or with dystonia. We had no idea how many people were going to show up for that first meeting. We must have done a good job of spreading the word about the support group because there were fourteen people with Parkinson's as well as their caregivers who came to the first meeting.

The fellow from Akron I had talked with while I was considering the procedure had started a group in his area and called his group "The Live Wires." With his permission we decided to call our group the same thing and we were off and running. Our first meeting was a get-to-know-you session with each of us telling our story. The group decided to meet once a month; I was thrilled that we were going to continue. I remember especially one lady who had read a little about DBS and was scared to death of the surgery. She said she was excited that I was doing so well but she just didn't think she could go through with it. It was three or four years after this meeting that she had the surgery and was very pleased with the outcome.

Another person was diagnosed with severe dystonia. She had been to a number of doctors who tried everything under the sun, moon, and stars but to no avail. She finally heard about DBS from her neurologist and eventually had the surgery. She was doing so well she claimed it was a miracle.

Another gentleman in the group had been diagnosed with essential tremor and had already had the surgery. He turned his system off and began to tremor almost uncontrollably. When he turned the stimulators back on, his tremors stopped immediately. It was an amazing demonstration.

The Live Wires group continued to meet for about two years and then it kind of fell apart. It wasn't that people weren't interested; it was a matter of age. The people just couldn't come any more. We did decide to stay in touch with each other by phone and email. Thank goodness for technology.

Dr. R moved his practice from the Cleveland Clinic to The Ohio State Medical Center in the spring of 2010. What a fortuitous move for me. Columbus is only an hour-and-a-half from home, whereas Cleveland is about four hours. So I transferred my care back to The Ohio State Medical Center where my PD journey had all started in 1988. My battery from the first surgery was beginning to wear out so my new programmer in Columbus said I should have it replaced in the fall. Dr. R agreed to do the surgery and he replaced the battery with a rechargeable one. The new battery would last about nine years as opposed to three to four years for the original battery. As he explained, the less often he had to do surgery the better to avoid infections. The new battery would need to be charged every week to a week and a half. That entailed sitting still for up to an hour with this round "antenna" held over the stimulator. Sitting still for an hour was and still is a real challenge for me. The other trick is to keep the antenna exactly in the right place for the hour.

The other battery needed to be replaced about six months or so after the first one was replaced. The longevity of the newer battery was better than the older one so I decided to go with the conventional (non-rechargeable) battery. I couldn't imagine sitting still enough to hold both chargers in the right place.

In the next chapter I will talk about life after the second surgery. This period (2007 to 2014) was pretty uneventful as far as the Parkinson's is concerned. People were amazed that I have had Parkinson's as long as I've had it. In December of 2013 I "celebrated" twenty-five years since my initial diagnosis by Dr. P. There have been so many opportunities during my retirement which have presented themselves enriching my life. It took a long time but I have come to the conclusion that Parkinson's is a blessing for me and my supportive family and for our six children, Greg, Geoff, Mark, Matt, Sarah, and Mary.

CHAPTER 6
THE PAST EIGHT YEARS

During the period of the last eight years, I continued to get phone calls from people wanting information about deep brain stimulation and Parkinson's in general. One experience especially stands out. I got a call from friends asking if I would talk to B who had been diagnosed approximately five years ago. I said yes and B called me from his summer place in northern Michigan. He wanted me to come to Michigan so he could meet me. Our friends also had a summer house next door to B and his wife which is how our friends had met this couple.

So, we picked a weekend and I drove up to northern Michigan. It was about an eight-hour drive from our house. I met B and we hit it off immediately. B decided to have the surgery (also at the Cleveland Clinic) and was very happy with the results. He was a retired dentist and after the surgery he became an unretired golfer. He loved the game and before the surgery couldn't play at all.

One of the major symptoms of Parkinson's that is not helped by the DBS surgery is the problem of poor balance. Falling became a big concern. Most people with Parkinson's report numerous falls, some more serious than others. I remember two falls in particular. The first one was while I was painting the kitchen. I was standing on a chair looking up, when I lost my balance and went over backwards with a loud crashing noise. Fortunately I didn't get hurt, but one of the chair rungs was smashed. After that little episode Judy wouldn't let me climb on a chair, ladder, or stepstool (aw, too bad!).

A couple of years later I was in the bathroom changing into my pajamas when my foot got tangled up the waistband of the pj's. I fell over on my left side between the bathtub and the toilet. I heard a crack when I landed and immediately knew I had broken a bone. It turned out to be that large bone that's connected to the hip. It didn't hurt, but I couldn't move my leg nor could I get up. So Judy called 911 and within a few minutes the ambulance and fire truck showed up at our door. They hoisted me up onto their hard (very hard) plastic stretcher and took me to the emergency room of our local hospital. There an x-ray confirmed a clean break of that large bone. Surgery was scheduled for the next afternoon to put a pin, rod, and two screws into the bone. I tried to tell the ambulance drivers that I should go for a helicopter ride to the hospital where my orthopedic surgeon practiced since it was about thirty miles from home, but they declined saying it was not a life threatening injury (too bad, as I've always wanted to go for a helicopter ride). What I did learn from this little episode was that I now put my pj's, pants, and undershorts on or off sitting on a chair or the bed.

I also learned that going to a rehab center which was part of a nursing home was not my idea of a whole lot of fun. They told me that I would need to stay in the nursing home for at least a month or until I could transfer in and out of a shower, in and out of a chair, and walk around the house with a walker. Their concern was that if I fell again Judy would be unable to pick me up. And so the challenge was on. The PT and OT sessions at least once a day were brutal. Finally, I met the criteria for going home in two-and-a-half weeks, not a month. Whenever I was supposed to do ten minutes on the exercise bike, I would do fifteen. Or when they told me to do ten reps of leg flexion, I would do fifteen. You get the picture. I was determined to beat their time frame.

When they released me from the rehab/nursing home I had PT and OT on an in-home basis. The therapists came about three times per week to continue the torture sessions (I mean the therapy sessions). As the weeks went by, it got easier and easier. I then graduated to outpatient therapy at the local hospital. In about two weeks of therapy I was able to walk without a cane. I felt as though I had joined the land of the living again.

I remember one particular session at home with the OT. She was testing me on activities of daily living. One of the items on her list was washing dishes. I told her that was no problem; I just put them into the dishwasher and turn it on. It was rather hilarious as she watched me do this little task. What sneaky way to get me to do the dishes!

By the end of April I was pretty much back to normal. I did not have full range of motion yet, but I was able to do about anything I did before the accident. What amazed me the most throughout this whole ordeal was the lack of pain. Sure, my muscles were sore after the PT sessions, but I was not in any pain whatsoever. The nurses at the hospital and nursing home kept trying to give me pain pills and I kept telling them that I did not need them.

In the fall of 2010 I was afforded the wonderful opportunity to become a research advocate with the Parkinson's Disease Foundation located in New York City. This is a national organization whose mission is to promote research toward finding a cure and discovering better treatment for symptoms. The whole idea is that the more people with Parkinson's enter into clinical trials, the more chances there are that we will eventually find a cure. We spent three full days in New Jersey at a workshop learning all about clinical trials, how to access research projects, and how to promote awareness of Parkinson's disease.

Another major goal of the organization is to promote awareness of the disease. There were about fifty people with Parkinson's going through the training which consisted of three full days of lectures from scientists who were conducting clinical trials. There were also members of the 2009 class who spent time teaching some of the things they did to promote awareness activities in their home cities and states. Some of the examples they gave were how to work with the media, putting up displays in the local libraries, and 5k races with special Parkinson's t-shirts.

For me it was exciting to be around and interact with other people who have Parkinson's. As we listened to each other's stories, we really got a sense of how wide a range of people were in the same boat. There was also a sense of similarity of symptoms and experiences.

Our "class" consisted of fifty people and was the second group that was trained. Our class brought the number of trainees to 100 working in approximately twenty-three states. Another aspect of the training was learning how to organize and operate support groups. Support groups are a prime target for signing up people to become involved in clinical trials. The PD Foundation developed a power point presentation covering the whole range of clinical trials. The most important aspect of the slide show was the point that if people chose not to participate in clinical trials we would never be able to find a cure or secure better options for symptom control.

One of the major roles of the Foundation is to encourage state-of-the-art research through its grants programs. For the past two years I had been involved in the summer fellowship grants program. These grants are awarded to students of all levels of university training who are doing basic research in a lab under the guidance of a mentor and professor. In 2013 there were approximately forty-five applications and we could fund between ten and fifteen grants at around $3,000 per grant. Our job was to review each grant application and then rank the grants with a recommendation for which ones to fund. I did not completely understand the science behind the research, but the Foundation wanted my input into which grants made the most sense for someone with Parkinson's disease. There were three of us "Parkies" reviewing the grants independently, and we came up with the same recommendations for which ones we should fund. That told me that the criteria were well put together and defined. Overall it was a great process. The level of the research ideas and the intelligence of the students were incredible. The main idea behind this grant program was to encourage students to go into Parkinson's research when they finished either their masters or doctoral programs.

A second grant program of the foundation was the international grant program. These were projects that were being conducted by established scientists. There were fifty-five grant applications with twelve to be funded (the total funding allocated was $1 million). Again there were very tight criteria. The funds for these projects were obtained through donations and fundraising activities nationwide.

The process for choosing the grant recipients entailed a detailed review of each of the fifty-five requests. The list was pared down to fifteen through an exhausting examination of each proposal by a number of the preeminent scientists who are presently involved in Parkinson's disease research. Those fifteen were then assigned to another group of scientists for a further in-depth review. The next step was to bring these people into the Foundation's office in New York City to finalize the accepted proposals. I was also invited to New York City to represent those who have Parkinson's. There were two people with Parkinson's and one caregiver in the room. I was one of the people with Parkinson's deliberating on each of the final proposals. Our role was to evaluate the relevance of each proposal from the perspective of someone who has Parkinson's disease. It was exciting to be part of a process that allowed input from people with Parkinson's to the final ranking of each proposal.

The next chapter is written by my wife Judy and will talk about the role of a care partner.

CHAPTER 7
ROLE OF A CARE PARTNER

By Judy Zimmerman

We need to grant them dignity and respect for who they are. As a care partner we, in turn, can learn so much from the person dealing with the numerous physical impairments of Parkinson's disease.

Forty years and six kids ago Bob and I said our "yeses" very loudly and clearly to our wedding vows.
"In sickness and in health…" "Yes." Of course. We are both healthy. No problem.
"For better or worse…" "Yes." Again, no problem.

What optimism! Little did we know that Bob would be diagnosed with Parkinson's disease at age forty-two, plus develop three different cancers, plus have a long recovery from a broken hip in the last ten years. Don't get me wrong. I would still have said my "Yes" just as loudly and clearly if I had known what was coming. After all Bob is the same person now (only better), but just in a somewhat damaged shell.

It is a privilege to be Bob's care partner. Except for the cancers and broken hip, his need for a care partner has been minimal. This is due in part to the great fortune of the slow progression of his disease. His amazingly positive attitude, his determination to not let this disease conquer him, his exercise routine and our generally healthy lifestyle have also contributed to his independence, as well as the support of family and friends.

Our kids, extended families and friends have become TEAM BOB cheerleaders. Our kids were ages two to twelve and all the even numbers between when Bob was diagnosed, so they have dealt with this disease for a long time also. It is fascinating to watch the role reversal they now evidence. They try to be inconspicuous as they walk closely beside their dad in case an unexpected crack in the sidewalk or curb shows up. They sandwich him between two of them as they climb steps at a Reds baseball game. Mary, who is an occupational therapist, has made numerous suggestions about easier methods for getting out of a car or chair and about furniture arrangement in our home. Mark engaged Bob in brewing beer during a recent visit in California. Greg and Geoff keep a ready supply of book suggestions for him. Matt and Sarah research herbs and foods and exercise routines to keep him healthy. The first question when friends and family call is, "How's Bob doing?" Even my ninety-five-year-old, four-foot-ten inch tall, 100 pound mom walks beside him ready to catch him if he loses his balance. So, my first suggestion is to allow and welcome the involvement of family and friends and accept their offers to help in their own way.

I have become a vigilante—always on the alert for danger from a slippery throw rug in someone's home or ice on the driveway or an upcoming step or curb. I request when we visit others that they keep pets away from where Bob is to prevent tripping over a sleeping cat or having a loss of balance from a bump by a dog. I scan ahead for possibilities of any seemingly innocent thing that could be a hazard for him. I am always searching for more efficient ways for Bob to do things like turning the handle of the milk carton to the outside to grab more easily or using a larger spoon to eat soup or using a cane to help get out of a low chair (some may call this nagging).

It has been very helpful for me to understand what Bob is dealing with and to learn the best ways to assist him by reading Parkinson's newsletters, doing research on line, and going to conferences with him. There are a lot of aha moments when learning more about the multiple physical repercussions of the disease. It helps to know, for example, that the sense of taste is diminished as well as smell so foods need to be seasoned a bit more. It helps to understand that swallowing can become a problem and drinking with a straw strengthens the muscles needed. Just little tips to make things easier and better for him. The knowledge helps me to do a better job.

Bob mentioned in an earlier chapter but I want to reemphasize the importance of accompanying him to doctor appointments. It is amazing even with both of us listening closely, while I take notes, how different our perceptions can be of what was said. It also helps the doctor to hear our observations of what is going on and problems occurring. As with all appointments it is essential to have a prepared list of questions before going to an appointment. It also helps me to feel more involved in Bob's treatment.

As a care partner it is very easy to develop a bad case of "poor me." Sure, I would have enjoyed taking a long hike in the jungle in Costa Rica (as long as snakes were not involved). It would have been wonderful to enjoy a sunset walk at Myrtle Beach. And oh how nice it would be to have help digging up the garden or washing walls. But better to think about what we *can* do together. After all, Bob is one who has to really deal with the limitations and it isn't his fault we can't do some things. So this means I often need an attitude adjustment.

A care partner needs to allow the person to be as independent as possible. This statement is probably in every pamphlet or book about rules for a care partner. This can be a tough one. I am a high energy person who likes to do things quickly and efficiently. Of course it would be much quicker for me to butter the toast or fold the laundry. But I cannot take that independence from Bob. It is important that he continues to do all he can at his own speed and in his own way. I cannot become an enabler. Independence definitely trumps efficiency and speed.

We care partners need to take care of ourselves. That also is in every pamphlet. We need to make time to exercise and meet with friends. We need to do things we enjoy. It is impossible to be a cheerleader and giver when we are emotionally and physically depleted. We also need to forgive ourselves for the very human and inevitable outbreaks of impatience and frustration.

Being a care partner is a two-way street. I have learned so much about patience and determination from Bob. I have developed so much respect for him as he persists with his exercises and deals with loss of balance (as a former coordinated athlete this is hard for him, so I need to be empathetic). His positive attitude is a trait every person should adopt. I am learning to slow down and "smell the roses," as the saying goes. Being a care partner is a gift. It allows me to express my love and care in ways I never could have imagined or anticipated. It helps to make me a better person.

Our daughter Mary's definition of her career as an occupational therapist is *teaching skills necessary for the job of life.* I would change the word definition slightly to *assisting* with the *skills necessary for the job of life* as the definition for a care partner. Our job is to assure that our person afflicted with the disease lives the best life he or she can with our help and support. We are cheerleaders.

CHAPTER 8
PRESENT

In the fall of 2013 I became aware of an exercise program which has proven to be effective in delaying the disease. Research studies have actually shown that the progression of the disease is slowed down. The two programs are called "THINK BIG" and "THINK LOUD." The THINK BIG program is a specific set of exercises that train the body to take big steps instead of the small shuffling steps. The exercises also aid in maintaining good posture and as a result, better balance. The THINK LOUD program is meant to train the person's voice to speak loudly rather than with a quiet voice. The THINK BIG program has also significantly improved my balance.

I learned that the physical therapy and the speech therapy departments at our local community hospital have therapists who are trained and certified in these programs. After doing some more research, I discovered that my health insurance would cover all the sessions. The only thing I needed was a prescription from my neurologist. So at my next scheduled appointment I asked Dr. S for the prescription for both programs. She said that I would be a perfect candidate for both programs.

I called my local community hospital and we set up the appointments for the first week in January, 2014. I was to go four days a week for four weeks. Each session was to last one hour for the speech program and one hour for the physical therapy program. The therapists did a pre-test to establish a baseline before the programs started. I was also told to do the specific routine of exercises every night at home. This was meant to develop the habit of thinking BIG and LOUD all of the time. I have to admit that by the time I got home after each session I was a whooped puppy. I did do my exercises each night at home as prescribed by the program.

At the end of the four weeks we did a post test and I was amazed at how much better I did on all the items tested. Improvement in my balance was the most significant item. I couldn't be more pleased with the outcomes of both programs. I would heartily recommend these programs for anyone with Parkinson's disease. Mr. Z also has a similar program called "Delay the Disease." He has put out a DVD which demonstrates very similar kinds of exercises.

At present I am on minimal amounts of medication. I take three 50mg of Sinemet daily and one 300mg of Wellbutrin, also daily. Wellbutrin is a mild anti-depressant which helps me get moving in the mornings. There are times during the day I forget to take the Sinemet pill, but I can't notice any difference. The "on-off" effect simply is not an issue. Dr. S suggested that I skip the evening dose for a week and if that makes no difference, I should skip the noon dose of Sinemet. And if that makes no difference, I should not take the morning dose. ALLELUIA!!! I would only be taking one pill a day.

Orthostatic hypotension has been a problem for a couple of years. This condition is the result of low blood pressure. So low at times that I get dizzy. When I sit down, the dizziness goes away. Usually this occurs in the mornings. But I think we have that problem licked. First, Dr. S suggested that I drink a minimum of a gallon of water a day. Second, I started drinking sixteen ounces of water before getting out of bed in the morning. Third, I should drink a cup of coffee in the morning to take advantage of the caffeine. And fourth, I should try wearing a pair of ted hose (compression hose that I have to fight to get on). These routines have helped tremendously. I have not been dizzy and my blood pressure has gone up to what's par for the course for me.

CONCLUSION
FINAL THOUGHTS

It is extremely frightening to get a diagnosis of Parkinson's disease. Most of the time there are some symptoms prior to actually getting the diagnosis. In my case I knew something was wrong with me almost a year before I went to my family physician. When I was actually diagnosed in December, 1988, I was shocked to say the least. When faced with the unknown, my wife and I began our quest for more information about Parkinson's disease. We read and read and then read some more from every source we could find. We literally became experts, as I mentioned.

My hope and reason for writing this book is for the newly diagnosed or for people who are just beginning their research to be encouraged and to understand that their lifestyle doesn't end with a diagnosis. This book is intended to give the reader my personal experiences with Parkinson's over the last twenty-six years of living with the disease. My hope is that some of the practical suggestions will help others cope with the disease and help, comfort, and receive encouragement from it. Keeping a notebook with all the information is really a key to helping the doctors remember from appointment to appointment what his or her long range treatment plan is for the Parkinson's patient.

Regular exercise is another crucial aspect of staying ahead of the disease process. As I've said, there is much research that now shows unequivocally that the patient can delay the progression of the disease with exercises such as those suggested by THIK BIG and THINK LOUD. Or, some find it refreshing to go for a walk for about thirty minutes a day. If one lives near a YMCA, water aerobics can be an excellent way to get daily exercise.

Hopefully if the reader only gets one little tidbit from this book, it will be that he or she must choose to have a positive attitude. My line is always that I refuse to let this disease intimidate me. There are so many things to do and see in this world, that we cannot let this disease stop us from enjoying them. So for one more time, rule #1 is keep a positive attitude.

When I was diagnosed twenty-six years ago, I set a goal for myself that I would walk down the church aisle at my two daughters' weddings. That dream came true in October, 2014, when our youngest daughter Mary married her high school sweetheart Scott. Besides walking with her down the aisle, I was also able to dance the traditional father-daughter dance at their reception. The best thing of all was that I did it without the use of a cane, walker, or wheelchair. Even better, I did not trip, stumble, or fall!